No Sugar for 30 Days

A Simple Plan to Improve Your Metabolism, Weight, and Blood Sugar Levels

Virgie W. Miller

COPYRIGHT

TABLE OF CONTENTS

INTRODUCTION

CHAPTER 1

 WHAT IS A SUGAR-FREE DIET, AND WHAT ARE THE HEALTH BENEFITS?

What is a diet without sugar?

What kinds of sugar are there, and how can they impact your health?

How does a sugar-free diet affect your blood sugar, weight, and metabolism?

Empirical support for a sugar-free diet

CHAPTER 2

 WHAT TO EAT AND AVOID AND HOW TO BEGIN A SUGAR-FREE DIET

How to eliminate sugar additives from your diet

Foods to include and exclude from a sugar-free diet

CHAPTER 3

HOW TO HANDLE SUGAR CRAVINGS AND SYMPTOMS OF WITHDRAWAL

What are the signs of sugar withdrawal and cravings?

How can I handle cravings for sugar and the symptoms of withdrawal?

CHAPTER 4

MAKING A SUGAR-FREE DIET A WAY OF LIFE RATHER THAN A PASSING TREND

Why avoiding sugar is a way of life rather than a passing trend

How to stick to a sugar-free diet in various circumstances

CHAPTER 5

RECIPES AND MEAL PLAN FOR NO-SUGAR DIET

An example 30-day sugar-free diet menu

Sugar-free diet recipes

CONCLUSION

INTRODUCTION

There is sugar all around us. It may be found in bread, sauces, snacks, beverages, and desserts. The sweet flavor and the quick energy boost it provides make it difficult to refuse. However, sugar is also among the greatest threats to our well-being. Inflammation, diabetes, heart disease, weight gain, and several other issues may be brought on by it. It may also lead to dependency, addiction, and unhappiness.

I decided to give up sweets for 30 days to test this out. In addition to wanting to feel better psychologically and emotionally. I wanted to know what my sugar intake was, how it affected me, and how I might survive without it.

I'll share my month-long sugar-free journey with you in this book. I'll share with you the things I discovered, went through, and accomplished. I'll also provide you with some pointers and counsel on how you may follow suit. You will learn about the advantages of a sugar-free diet, the obstacles and problems associated with giving up sugar, and the methods and solutions to get through them. Along with some delectable and simple dishes you can attempt at home, you will also receive a sample 30-day no-sugar diet meal plan.

This book is not a hard diet regimen that you must adhere to precisely. You may modify this easy-to-use guide to suit your tastes and requirements. Furthermore, it's not a tasteless, monotonous diet that robs you of flavor and pleasure. You may indulge in your sweet appetite with natural alternatives while following this enjoyable and fulfilling diet that lets you consume a wide range of foods.

Join me in this no-sugar challenge if you're prepared to take charge of your happiness and well-being and you'll be able to see the results for yourself. Sugar is the only thing you have to lose, and you stand to gain much. Now let's get going!

CHAPTER 1

WHAT IS A SUGAR-FREE DIET, AND WHAT ARE THE HEALTH BENEFITS?

What is a diet without sugar?

A no-sugar diet is a way of eating that attempts to cut down or completely exclude added sugar. Any kind of sugar that isn't found naturally in meals like fruit, vegetables, and dairy products is referred to as added sugar. Processed foods including candy, soda, cookies, cakes, ice cream, morning cereals, sauces, and condiments often include added sugar. The customer may also add it to meals and drinks, such as sugar in tea or coffee.

You do not have to abstain from all sugar to follow a no-sugar diet. Fruits, vegetables, dairy products, and other foods that naturally contain sugar may still be consumed since they are a good source of fiber and other nutrients. Foods rich in natural sugar, including fruit juice, honey, and dried fruit, should be consumed in moderation since they still have the potential to spike blood sugar levels and add unnecessary calories.

Reducing your consumption of empty calories—calories with no nutritional value—is the primary objective of a no-sugar diet, which aims to enhance your health. You may reduce your risk of obesity, diabetes, heart disease, and other chronic illnesses associated with excessive sugar intake by avoiding added sugar.

What kinds of sugar are there, and how can they impact your health?

One kind of carbohydrate, a macronutrient that gives your body energy, is sugar. Sugar comes in two primary forms: disaccharides and monosaccharides. Simple sugars with just one molecule, such as glucose, fructose, and galactose, are known as monosaccharides. Disaccharides, including lactose, maltose, and sucrose, are complex sugars made up of two molecules each.

The most prevalent kind of sugar and your cells' primary source of energy is glucose. Foods including wheat, potatoes, and legumes contain glucose. Fruit's sweet flavor is attributed to fructose, a kind of sugar. Moreover, high fructose corn syrup, a prevalent sweetener in processed foods, and honey both contain fructose. The sugar contained in milk and dairy products is called galactose.

Table sugar, which is produced from sugar cane or sugar beet, is known by its scientific name, sucrose. Glucose and fructose combine to form sucrose. The kind of sugar included in milk and dairy products is called lactose. Glucose and galactose make up lactose. The sugar that results from the breakdown of starch is called maltose. Two glucose molecules make up one maltose molecule.

All forms of sugar increase blood sugar levels because they are broken down and absorbed into the circulation. In response, your body releases the hormone insulin, which facilitates the uptake of glucose by your cells and its energy conversion. Insulin also instructs your body to store extra glucose as fat in your adipose tissue or as glycogen in your muscles and liver.

Consuming excessive amounts of sugar can be harmful to your health. Overindulgence in sugar may overwhelm your liver, causing it to convert fructose into fat and ultimately result in inflammation and fatty liver disease. Additionally, consuming too much sugar may alter your blood sugar levels and reduce your sensitivity to insulin, which can result in insulin resistance and type 2 diabetes. In addition to raising your risk of heart disease and stroke, too much sugar may also raise your triglyceride and cholesterol levels.

How does a sugar-free diet affect your blood sugar, weight, and metabolism?

Your weight, blood sugar levels, and metabolism may all benefit from a no-sugar diet. By consuming less added sugar, you can:

- Reduce your caloric intake and avoid overindulging. Added sugar does not make you feel full or quell your appetite since it is heavy in calories and lacking in nutrients and satiety. You may lower your calorie intake and steer clear of pointless eating and bingeing by avoiding added sugar.
- Boost your blood sugar regulation and insulin sensitivity. Your blood sugar levels may surge and fall as a result of added sugar, which may reduce your sensitivity to insulin and increase your risk of developing diabetes and insulin

resistance. Eliminating added sugar may help you manage or avoid diabetes and its problems by stabilizing your blood sugar levels and enhancing your insulin sensitivity.

- Lower your chance of cardiovascular disease and metabolic syndrome. Your triglyceride and cholesterol levels may rise as a result of added sugar, which may exacerbate metabolic syndrome and cardiovascular disease. A group of illnesses known as metabolic syndrome include elevated blood pressure, elevated blood sugar, extra belly fat, and abnormally high cholesterol. Heart attacks and strokes are examples of conditions that fall within the umbrella of cardiovascular disease. Eliminating added sugar lowers cholesterol and triglyceride levels, which in turn lowers the risk of metabolic syndrome and cardiovascular disease.

Empirical support for a sugar-free diet

Scientific data substantiates the health advantages of a sugar-free diet. Reducing or eliminating added sugar from your diet has been linked in many studies to better blood sugar regulation, decreased blood pressure, lower cholesterol, decreased inflammation, and weight reduction.

For instance, a randomized controlled experiment with forty-three obese children discovered that, without altering their calorie consumption or physical activity, substituting starch for added sugar for nine days led to substantial drops in blood pressure, blood sugar, insulin, and triglycerides.

Reducing added sugar intake from 28% to 10% of calories for 12 weeks resulted in significant weight loss, improved blood sugar control, lower blood pressure, lower cholesterol levels, and reduced inflammation, according to another randomized controlled trial involving 174 adults with obesity or overweight. The control group continued to consume sugar as usual.

Independent of body weight, a systematic review and meta-analysis of 37 trials comprising 405,907 people revealed that consuming more added sugar was linked to an elevated risk of type 2 diabetes.

Higher intake of added sugar was linked to an elevated risk of cardiovascular disease mortality, irrespective of body weight, physical activity, smoking, and alcohol use, according to a systematic review and meta-analysis of 39 studies comprising 176,310 people.

Unaffected by body weight or alcohol intake, a systematic review and meta-analysis of 68 trials with 907,957 individuals revealed that a greater intake of added sugar was linked to a higher risk of fatty liver disease.

These studies provide compelling proof that cutting off sugar may improve blood sugar regulation, weight management, and metabolism, and reduce the chance of developing chronic illnesses.

CHAPTER 2

WHAT TO EAT AND AVOID AND HOW TO BEGIN A SUGAR-FREE DIET

How to eliminate sugar additives from your diet

Although it might be difficult, eliminating additional sugar from your diet is not impossible. Here are some useful pointers and recommendations for cutting down on sugar consumption and choosing healthier options:

- Examine the food labels. Finding out where extra sugar lurks is the first step towards avoiding it. Bread, spaghetti sauce, salad dressing, ketchup, and yogurt are just a few examples of foods that may not immediately come to mind as sweet, yet they may contain substantial levels of added sugar. Look for terms like sucrose, glucose, fructose, maltose, honey, corn syrup, and molasses in the ingredients list. These are indicators of added sugar. For information on the total and added sugar content per serving, you may also refer to the nutrition facts label. Select meals with less than 5 grams of added sugar per 100 grams of food.

- Opt for whole foods. Whole foods are those that have undergone little processing and are almost unprocessed. Fruits, vegetables, legumes, nuts, seeds, eggs, meat, fish, and dairy products are among them. Whole foods often have little to no added sugar and are high in antioxidants, fiber, and minerals. Additionally, they aid in satiation and fullness, which might lessen cravings for sweets. Every meal, try to have non-starchy veggies take up at least half of your plate. You should also add a reasonable quantity of protein and healthy fats.

- Steer clear of processed meals. Foods that have been processed have changed from their original form, often by the addition of artificial tastes and colors, sugar, salt, fat, and preservatives. Candy, soda, cakes, cookies, ice cream, chips, crackers, cereals, and frozen dinners are some of them. Processed foods are heavy in calories and lacking in nutrients, which may increase hunger and lead to overindulgence. Additionally, they may cause blood sugar irregularities and raise your risk of heart disease, diabetes, and obesity. Reduce or cut out processed items from your diet in favor of homemade or fresh meals.

- Sip on water or other unsweetened drinks. Drinks make up around 25% of the added sugar consumed in the American diet, making them one of the primary sources of this sugar. Up to 10 teaspoons of sugar are included in a serving of soda, juice, sports drinks, energy drinks, and sweetened coffee and tea. These liquid calories build up fast, which may lead to health issues and weight gain. Drink water or unsweetened liquids like milk, coffee, herbal tea, black or green tea, or sparkling water to keep hydrated and healthy. For a cool twist, you may also add flavors to your water like lemon, cucumber, mint, or berries.

Foods to include and exclude from a sugar-free diet

You must be aware of which items to consume and which to avoid to adhere to a sugar-free diet. The following is a broad list of things that are excellent or harmful for you to eat or not eat when following a no-sugar diet:

Food items to eat

- Vegetables without starches. Leafy greens, broccoli, cauliflower, cabbage, celery, cucumber, zucchini, eggplant, mushrooms, peppers, tomatoes, and onions are examples of vegetables that are low in sugar and carbs. They may help reduce blood sugar levels and aid digestion since they are rich in fiber, vitamins, minerals, and antioxidants. They may be added to salads, soups, stir-fries, casseroles, and other dishes.They may be roasted, boiled, or eaten raw.

- **Fruits:** These fruits, which include berries, apples, pears, oranges, grapefruit, kiwi, melon, and peaches, have low to moderate sugar content. In addition to being abundant in fiber, vitamins, minerals, and antioxidants, they may help strengthen your immune system and sate your sweet craving. They may be added to smoothies, fruit salads, desserts, or eaten fresh, frozen, or dried. However, since they might boost your blood sugar levels and increase your calorie intake, restrict your consumption of fruits that are rich in sugar, such as grapes, bananas, mangoes, and pineapples.

- **Seeds and nuts:** These include foods like almonds, walnuts, pistachios, cashews, sunflower seeds, pumpkin seeds, chia seeds, and flax seeds that are high in protein, fiber, and healthy fats. They may help keep you full and pleased, reduce your cholesterol, and enhance cognitive performance. They may be added to granola, bars, and trail mixes, or eaten raw, roasted, or as nut butter. On the other hand, stay away from nuts and seeds that have been covered in chocolate, honey, or sugar since they might add extra calories and sugar to your diet.

- **Vegetables:** These include foods like beans, lentils, peas, and soy that are rich in iron, fiber, protein, and folate. They may improve the health of your heart and digestive systems and help decrease blood pressure, cholesterol, and blood sugar levels. They may be added to soups, salads, burgers, and hummus in addition to being eaten cooked, canned, or sprouted. On the other hand, stay away from sugar-prepared legumes like baked beans and sweetened soy products like yogurt or milk.

- **Eggs:** These are meals rich in healthy fats, protein, and choline, a vitamin vital to the functioning of your liver and brain. In addition to preventing muscle loss, eggs may help control blood sugar levels, metabolism, hunger, and metabolism. They may be added to quiches, frittatas, or muffins, or eaten boiled, scrambled, poached, or as omelets. On the other hand, stay away from frying eggs in butter or oil or combining them with sugar, such as in pancakes or waffles.

- **Fish and meat:** These are the kinds of meals that are good for your muscles, bones, immune system, and brain since they are rich in protein, iron, zinc, and omega-3 fatty acids. Meat and fish have been shown to reduce blood pressure and inflammation while also improving satiety, metabolism, and muscle mass. They go well with roasting, baking, and grilling. They may also be used for tacos, wraps, and sandwiches.

But stay away from processed, cured, or smoked meat and fish (such as bacon, ham, salami, sausages, or hot dogs) since they may have extra sugar, salt, or preservatives.

- **Products made from dairy**: These are foods that are good for your bones, teeth, muscles, and digestive system since they are rich in calcium, protein, and probiotics. Dairy products may strengthen your immune system, aid with digestion, and help prevent osteoporosis. They may be added to smoothies, dips, and sauces, or consumed as milk, cheese, yogurt, or cottage cheese. But stay away from flavored, sweetened, or low-fat dairy products like fruit yogurt, ice cream, or chocolate milk as they may have artificial flavors, fillers, and extra sugar.

Foods to stay away from

- **Sweeteners and sugar**: These meals may lead to weight gain, diabetes, heart disease, and other health issues since they are heavy in calories and lacking in nutrients. Table sugar, brown sugar, powdered sugar, honey, maple syrup, agave nectar, molasses, corn syrup, and artificial sweeteners including aspartame, sucralose, and saccharin are examples of sugar and sweeteners. Choose unsweetened or naturally sweetened alternatives to sugar and sweeteners while preparing meals and drinks.

- **Prepared meals**: These are foods that have undergone modifications from their original form, often by the addition of preservatives, artificial tastes and colors, sugar, salt, and fat. Candy, soda, cakes, cookies, ice cream, chips, crackers, cereals, and frozen dinners are some of them. Processed foods are heavy in calories and lacking in nutrients, which may increase hunger and lead to overindulgence. They may also raise your risk of obesity, diabetes, and heart disease, as well as interfere with your blood sugar levels. Reduce or completely cut out processed items from your diet in favor of homemade or fresh meals.

- **Grain refinement:** The bran and germ of the grains—which contain the majority of the fiber, vitamins, minerals, and antioxidants—have been removed from these grains. White crackers, white bread, white rice, white pasta, and white flour are among them. Refined grains may produce insulin spikes and elevated blood sugar levels since they are poor in fiber and rich in carbs. They may also intensify your appetites and hunger, which may result in overindulging and weight gain. Instead, choose for whole grains like buckwheat, quinoa, barley, oats, and whole wheat. These high-fiber, nutrient-dense foods may help control blood sugar levels and keep you feeling full and content.

- **Spirits**. This is a material that is created by the fermentation of yeast and sugar and is present in beverages including wine, beer, liquor, and cocktails. Alcohol may affect your metabolism and liver function. It is also poor in nutrients and heavy in calories. It may also impact insulin sensitivity and blood sugar levels, as well as heighten cravings and hunger. In addition, it may lead to headaches, dehydration, and poor sleep quality and mood. Drink little or no alcohol at all, and substitute water or other unsweetened liquids. If you do consume alcohol, choose low-sugar choices like diet tonic, light lager, or dry wine. You may also choose to drink in moderation by pairing spirits with soda water.

CHAPTER 3

HOW TO HANDLE SUGAR CRAVINGS AND SYMPTOMS OF WITHDRAWAL

What are the signs of sugar withdrawal and cravings?

Strong, compulsive desires to consume anything sweet are known as sugar cravings, and they are often brought on by emotions, stress, boredom, or hunger. Due to sugar's addictive properties, which activate our brain's pleasure and reward centers and produce the feel-good chemical dopamine, cravings for sugar are brought on. In addition to your behaviors, surroundings, and social cues—like smelling or seeing something sweet or having a friend offer you dessert—all have an impact on your need for sugar.

The physical and psychological side effects you could encounter while cutting down on sugar are known as sugar withdrawal symptoms. The symptoms of sugar withdrawal are brought on by changes in hormone levels and brain chemistry as well as your body's sugar detoxification process. Headaches, lethargy, irritability, mood changes, anxiety, melancholy, nausea, dizziness, and flu-like symptoms are some of the symptoms associated with sugar withdrawal. The severity and length of sugar withdrawal symptoms might vary based on personal characteristics including sugar consumption, metabolism, and health.

How can I handle cravings for sugar and the symptoms of withdrawal?

Overcoming sugar cravings and withdrawal symptoms might be difficult, but not impossible. To help you deal with them and maintain your no-sugar diet, consider the following tactics and solutions:

- Sip some water. Water may help you manage your sugar cravings and withdrawal symptoms in addition to being vital for your health and hydration. Water may assist your body in eliminating toxins, controlling blood sugar, and avoiding dehydration, which can lead to weariness and headaches. Additionally, drinking water helps satisfy your hunger and lessen your appetite.You should drink eight glasses of water or more every day. If you experience withdrawal symptoms or a sugar desire, sip a glass of water and wait fifteen minutes. Your symptom or desire may have lessened or vanished.

- Consume fruits. Fruits are nature's candy; in addition to providing you with nutrients and antioxidants, they may help you sate your sweet craving. Fruits include natural sugar, which is distinct from added sugar since they also contain fiber, vitamins, minerals, and phytochemicals that help reduce blood sugar rise and slow down the absorption of sugar. Fruits may also lower oxidative stress and inflammation while elevating your energy and happiness. When you're wanting sugar, grab a handful of berries or a piece of fruit; go for low- to moderate-sugar fruits like berries, apples, pears, oranges, grapefruit, kiwi, melon, and peaches.

- Work out. One of the greatest methods to manage sugar cravings and withdrawal symptoms is to exercise, as it helps produce endorphins, which are feel-good, naturally occurring chemicals that also help with pain and stress management. In addition to helping you burn fat and calories, exercise helps strengthen your immune system, metabolism, and blood circulation. Exercise may also make you feel accomplished and satisfied while diverting your attention from your symptoms and desires. Choose an activity you love and can maintain, such as walking, running, cycling, swimming, or dancing, and commit to at least 30 minutes of moderate to intense exercise each day.

- Take a moment to meditate. In meditation, you let go of your thoughts, emotions, and sensations and instead direct your attention to your breath, a word, a sound, or an object. Since meditation may relax your body and mind and lessen tension and anxiety, it can help you deal with sugar cravings and withdrawal symptoms. Additionally, meditation may help you become more alert and observant of your surroundings, as well as identify and withstand your symptoms and urges. Look for a peaceful, comfortable spot to sit or lie down and meditate for at least ten minutes each day, either in the morning or just before bed. To assist with meditation, you may also utilize a guided meditation app or video, or you can just listen to relaxing music or noises.

CHAPTER 4

MAKING A SUGAR-FREE DIET A WAY OF LIFE RATHER THAN A PASSING TREND

Why avoiding sugar is a way of life rather than a passing trend

A sugar-free diet is a way of life, not just a trend. A fad is a transient, popular diet that makes extravagant, speedy claims of outcomes but often falls short of being sustainable or long-lasting. A lifestyle is a consistent, healthful eating plan that may be tailored to your unique requirements and tastes while supporting your overall objectives and well-being.

A sugar-free diet is a way of life since it may enhance your weight, health, and overall quality of life. It is founded on solid scientific facts and principles. Through the reduction of inflammation, oxidative stress, and insulin resistance, a sugar-free diet may aid in the prevention or management of chronic conditions including diabetes, obesity, heart disease, and cancer. By balancing your blood sugar and neurotransmitter levels, a sugar-free diet may also improve your mood, energy, and mental clarity. A sugar-free diet may also increase your enjoyment of food by reprogramming your taste buds and heightening your sense of natural flavor.

A sugar-free diet is a lifelong habit rather than a short-term solution. A habit is an action that, with consistent repetition and reward, develops over time into a reflexive, easy behavior. A habit is also impacted by identity, signals, rewards, and surroundings. You must fit your environment, routine, and mentality with your beliefs and objectives to develop a no-sugar diet habit.

How to stick to a sugar-free diet in various circumstances

It may be difficult to stick to a sugar-free diet in a variety of contexts, including dining out, traveling, celebrating, and socializing. That is not difficult, however, provided you prepare yourself, have a flexible schedule, and plan beforehand. Here are some pointers and strategies for maintaining a sugar-free diet in various scenarios:

- **Dining out:** Dining out may be challenging since a lot of cafés and restaurants provide food and beverages that are poor in fiber and minerals and high in sugar, salt, and fat. To resist temptation and choose better options, you can:

- Look up the menu online before you go.. Look for low-sugar options like salads, soups, grilled meats, or seafood, and steer clear of high-sugar options like spaghetti, pizza, burgers, or sweets.

- Request adjustments or replacements, such as additional veggies, extra dressing, no cheese, or sauce; exclude extras like bread, chips, or drink.

- Rather than ordering from the menu, bring your desserts or snacks, such as nuts, fruits, or dark chocolate, and enjoy them after your dinner.

- Avoid sugary drinks like soda, juice, sports drinks, energy drinks, sweetened coffee, and tea, and instead stick to drinking water or unsweetened liquids like sparkling water, herbal tea, black or green tea, coffee, or milk.

- **Journeying**: when you experience new meals, timetables, and cultures when traveling, you can also experience stress since you won't always have access to your regular foods and habits. To maintain focus and have fun on your journey, you can:

- Bring your food on flights, trains, and automobiles. This way, you may eat when you're hungry rather than depending on the potentially unhealthy, high-sugar, high-fat alternatives that are offered. Examples of this food include nuts, seeds, dried fruits, granola bars, and sandwiches.

- When making your hotel selection, try to find a place with a kitchen, refrigerator, or microwave so you can cook for yourself or at least keep some fresh or frozen foods like cheese, yogurt, or fruits and use them for breakfast or snacks instead of going out to eat or getting room service.

- Selective eating is encouraged while exploring the local food. Low-sugar options include salads, soups, grilled meats, and fish. High-sugar options include pastries, cakes, ice cream, and candies. To add some taste and diversity to your diet, you may also experiment with some locally grown fruits, veggies, or spices that are rich in antioxidants and minerals.

- To stay hydrated and improve your mood and sleep quality, it is recommended that you drink plenty of water or unsweetened liquids like milk, sparkling water, herbal tea, black or green tea, coffee, or tea. Sugary drinks like soda, juice, sports drinks, energy drinks, or alcoholic beverages should be avoided.

- **Joyful:** Celebrating may be happy, but it can also be difficult since you can be exposed to more sugar-rich foods and beverages, such as cakes, cookies, chocolates, and cocktails, as well as peer pressure, social expectations, and emotional triggers. To maintain your health and have pleasure, you can:

  - Make a plan, establish limits, determine what and how much to eat and drink, follow through on your plan, and refrain from overindulging or bingeing. You may also tell your loved ones about your sugar-free diet, solicit their help and understanding, and steer clear of criticism or condemnation.

  - Bring your snacks or beverages, such as dark chocolate, almonds, fruits, or sparkling water, and enjoy them during the celebration rather than consuming the potentially high-sugar, high-fat food and beverages that are provided. Additionally, you may demonstrate to people that you can celebrate without sugar by sharing your snacks or beverages with them.

- Instead of depending on sugar to make you feel better or give you more energy, enjoy the conversation, music, games, dancing, the occasion, and the people around you instead of the food and drink. Without feeling bad about your decisions or regretting them, you may also show your appreciation and thanks to the host, the visitors, or the event and create some wonderful memories.

- **Making friends:** Socializing may be enjoyable but sometimes challenging since you may run across people with various beliefs, tastes, and routines. You may also face additional diversions and temptations and have less regularity and control over the meals and beverages you consume. To maintain your sugar-free diet and stay in touch, you can:

- Pick your locations and activities wisely. Go for low-sugar alternatives like bicycling, hiking, bowling, or movies; stay away from high-sugar ones like bars, parties, and buffets. Additionally, you may recommend or decide on eateries that provide delectable and healthful fare like salads, soups, grilled meats, fish, and beverages like milk, tea, coffee, or tea. On the other hand, you should stay away from eateries that serve sugary and unhealthy fare like pizza, burgers, fries, and soda.

- Say goodbye to sugar-laden meals and beverages and be strong and forceful in your approach. Don't hesitate to share the reasons for your sugar-free diet and its advantages. You may even accept sugar-free goods and beverages as long as you praise their flavor, quality, or appearance. Without passing judgment or offering criticism, you may also learn more about other people's tastes and habits by enquiring about and demonstrating an interest in the meals and beverages they are consuming.

 - Be practical and adaptable, and sometimes give yourself certain pleasures and exceptions. Then, enjoy them guilt-free. To maintain your general health and weight, you may also balance them with some moderation and compensation, eat or drink less or more of anything else, or exercise more or less. To make your no-sugar diet more enduring and pleasurable, you may also incorporate lessons learned from your errors and experiences into your plan and approach.

CHAPTER 5

RECIPES AND MEAL PLAN FOR NO-SUGAR DIET

An example 30-day sugar-free diet menu

Having a meal plan that tells you what to eat and when might make sticking to a sugar-free diet simpler and more fun. In addition to helping you prevent food waste and temptation, a meal plan may help you save time, money, and energy. This is an example 30-day no-sugar diet menu that you may use as a model or change to fit your requirements and tastes. The daily meal plan delivers around 1,500 calories and consists of breakfast, lunch, supper, and two snacks. You may modify the serving sizes and caloric content to meet your specific needs and objectives.

Day1

- One cup of oatmeal, one cup of low-fat milk, one apple, and cinnamon for breakfast.

- One small banana with two spoonfuls of almond butter for a morning snack

- Lunch consists of 2 whole-wheat slices, 3 ounces of turkey, ¼ avocado, sliced tomato, and 1 cup of greens.

- Snack in the afternoon: 1 cup sugar snap peas and bell peppers with 1 stick of mozzarella cheese

- Dinner consists of one dish of shrimp and avocado pesto over zucchini noodles.[3]

Day 2

- Two scrambled eggs, two pieces of whole-wheat bread, and one cup of strawberries for breakfast

- 1/4 cup mixed nuts and 1 clementine as a morning snack

- Lunch: A single plate of Parmesan vinaigrette-topped spinach and artichoke salad[3]

- Snack in the afternoon: 1/4 cup granola, 1/2 cup plain Greek yogurt, and 1/4 cup blueberries

- One dish of beef chili in an instant pot with sweet potatoes for dinner.

Day 3

- Breakfast: One muffin-tin mini-quiche with spinach and mushrooms[4]- One serving of Peanut Butter-Date Energy Balls for breakfast- Lunch consists of one plate of parmesan vinaigrette-topped spinach and artichoke salad.[2]- Snack in the afternoon: 1/2 cup of grapes and 1 hard-boiled egg

The supper consists of one dish of roasted salmon, smoked chickpeas, and greens.

Day 4

- Breakfast: One muffin-tin mini-quiche with spinach and mushrooms[4]

- 1/4 cup hummus with 1 whole-wheat pita bread and 1/2 cup cherry tomatoes for a morning snack.

- Lunch: A single plate of Parmesan vinaigrette-topped spinach and artichoke salad[2] - Snack in the afternoon: 1/4 cup raspberries with 1/2 cup cottage cheese

- One dish of brown rice and stir-fried chicken and vegetables for dinner.

Day 5

- Breakfast consists of 1/4 cup granola, 1/4 cup blueberries, and 1 cup plain Greek yogurt.

- One pear and one ounce of cheddar cheese for breakfast

- Lunch: A single plate of Parmesan vinaigrette-topped spinach and artichoke salad[2]- Snack in the afternoon: One dish of Peanut Butter-Date Energy Balls[5]- One dish of Mediterranean Quinoa Salad for dinner

Day 6

- Breakfast: One muffin-tin mini-quiche with spinach and mushrooms ♨

- 1/4 cup mixed nuts and 1 clementine as a morning snack

- One dish of Mediterranean Quinoa Salad for lunch

- Snack in the afternoon: 1/4 cup granola, 1/2 cup plain Greek yogurt, and 1/4 cup blueberries

- One bowl of black bean soup for dinner

Day 7

- Two scrambled eggs, two pieces of whole-wheat bread, and one cup of strawberries for breakfast

One small banana and two spoonfuls of almond butter for a morning snack; one bowl of black bean soup for lunch

- Snack in the afternoon: 1 cup sugar snap peas and bell peppers plus 1 stick of mozzarella cheese - Dinner: 1 dish of baked chicken with a nut crust and garlicky green beans

Day 8

- One cup of oatmeal, one cup of low-fat milk, one apple, and cinnamon for breakfast.

- 1/4 cup hummus with 1 whole-wheat pita bread and 1/2 cup cherry tomatoes for a morning snack.

Lunch consists of 2 whole-wheat slices, 3 ounces of tuna, 1 tablespoon of mayonnaise, 1/4 cup of celery, and 1 cup of greens.

- Snack in the afternoon: 1/4 cup raspberries with 1/2 cup cottage cheese

- One dish of spaghetti for dinner Squash Pasta

Day 9

- Two scrambled eggs, two pieces of whole-wheat bread, and one cup of strawberries for breakfast

- One serving of Peanut Butter-Date Energy Balls for breakfast[5]

- One dish of spaghetti squash spaghetti for lunch

Snack in the afternoon: 1/2 cup of grapes and one hard-boiled egg.

- Supper: One dish of shrimp scampi

Day 10

- Breakfast consists of 1/4 cup granola, 1/4 cup blueberries, and 1 cup plain Greek yogurt.

- One pear and one ounce of cheddar cheese for breakfast

- Lunch: One dish of pasta salad with avocado.

- Snack in the afternoon: 1/4 cup mixed nuts with 1 clementine

- Supper is one dish of citrus celery salad.

Day 11

- Breakfast: One muffin-tin mini-quiche with spinach and mushrooms ♨

- 1/4 cup hummus with 1 whole-wheat pita bread and 1/2 cup cherry tomatoes for a morning snack.

- Lunch: One dish of celery and citrus salad

- Snack in the afternoon: 1/4 cup granola, 1/2 cup plain Greek yogurt, and 1/4 cup blueberries
- Supper is one dish of white rice and dill carrots

Day 12

- One cup of oatmeal, one cup of low-fat milk, one apple, and cinnamon for breakfast.
- One small banana with two spoonfuls of almond butter for a morning snack
- Lunch consists of 2 whole-wheat slices, 3 ounces of chicken, 1/4 cup pesto, sliced tomato, and 1 cup of greens.
- Snack in the afternoon: 1 cup sugar snap peas and bell peppers with 1 stick of mozzarella cheese
The supper consists of one dish of roasted salmon, smoked chickpeas, and greens.

Day 13

- Two scrambled eggs, two pieces of whole-wheat bread, and one cup of strawberries for breakfast

- One serving of Peanut Butter-Date Energy Balls for breakfast[5]

- Lunch consists of one dish of roasted salmon, smoked chickpeas, and greens.

Snack in the afternoon: 1/2 cup of grapes and one hard-boiled egg.

- One dish of brown rice and stir-fried chicken and vegetables for dinner.

Day 14

- Morning snack: 1 pear + 1 oz cheddar cheese

- Breakfast: 1 cup plain Greek yogurt + 1/4 cup granola + 1/4 cup blueberries

- Lunch: 1 dish of stir-fried chicken and vegetables-Saute over brown rice

- Snack in the afternoon: 1/4 cup mixed nuts with 1 clementine
- One dish of Mediterranean Quinoa Salad for dinner

Day 15

- Breakfast: One muffin-tin mini-quiche with spinach and mushrooms ♨
- 1/4 cup hummus with 1 whole-wheat pita bread and 1/2 cup cherry tomatoes for a morning snack.
- One dish of Mediterranean Quinoa Salad for lunch
- Snack in the afternoon: 1/4 cup raspberries with 1/2 cup cottage cheese
- One bowl of black bean soup for dinner

Day 16

- One cup of oatmeal, one cup of low-fat milk, one apple, and cinnamon for breakfast.

- One small banana with two spoonfuls of almond butter for a morning snack

- Lunch is one bowl of black bean soup.

- Snack in the afternoon: 1 cup sugar snap peas and bell peppers with 1 stick of mozzarella cheese

- Dinner consists of one dish of baked chicken with nut crust and garlicky green beans.

Day 17

- Two scrambled eggs, two pieces of whole-wheat bread, and one cup of strawberries for breakfast

- One serving of Peanut Butter-Date Energy Balls for breakfast[5]

- Lunch consists of 2 pieces of whole-wheat bread, 3 ounces of ham, 1 slice of cheese, 1 teaspoon of mustard, and 1 cup of greens.

Snack in the afternoon: 1/2 cup of grapes and one hard-boiled egg.

- One dish of spaghetti squash spaghetti for dinner

Day 18

- Breakfast consists of 1/4 cup granola, 1/4 cup blueberries, and 1 cup plain Greek yogurt.

- One pear and one ounce of cheddar cheese for breakfast

- One dish of spaghetti squash spaghetti for lunch

- Snack in the afternoon: 1/4 cup mixed nuts with 1 clementine

- Supper: One dish of shrimp scampi

Day 19

- Breakfast: One muffin-tin mini-quiche with spinach and mushrooms

- 1/4 cup hummus with 1 whole-wheat pita bread and 1/2 cup cherry tomatoes for a morning snack.

- One dish of shrimp scampi for lunch

- Snack in the afternoon: 1/4 cup granola, 1/2 cup plain Greek yogurt, and 1/4 cup blueberries The supper consists of one dish of roasted salmon, smoked chickpeas, and greens.

Day 20

- One cup of oatmeal, one cup of low-fat milk, one apple, and cinnamon for breakfast.

- One small banana with two spoonfuls of almond butter for a morning snack

- Lunch consists of one dish of roasted salmon, smoked chickpeas, and greens.

- Snack in the afternoon: 1 cup sugar snap peas and bell peppers with 1 stick of mozzarella cheese
- One dish of brown rice and stir-fried chicken and vegetables for dinner.

Day 21

- Two scrambled eggs, two pieces of whole-wheat bread, and one cup of strawberries for breakfast
- One serving of Peanut Butter-Date Energy Balls for breakfast
- Lunch is one dish of brown rice and stir-fried chicken and vegetables.
Snack in the afternoon: 1/2 cup of grapes and one hard-boiled egg.
- One dish of Mediterranean Quinoa Salad for dinner

Day 22

- Breakfast consists of 1/4 cup granola, 1/4 cup blueberries, and 1 cup plain Greek yogurt.

- One pear and one ounce of cheddar cheese for breakfast

- One dish of Mediterranean Quinoa Salad for lunch

- Snack in the afternoon: 1/4 cup mixed nuts with 1 clementine

- One bowl of black bean soup for dinner

Day 23

- Breakfast: One muffin-tin mini-quiche with spinach and mushrooms

- 1/4 cup hummus with 1 whole-wheat pita bread and 1/2 cup cherry tomatoes for a morning snack.

- Lunch is one bowl of black bean soup.

- Snack in the afternoon: 1/4 cup raspberries with 1/2 cup cottage cheese

- Dinner consists of one dish of baked chicken with nut crust and garlicky green beans.

Day 24

- One cup of oatmeal, one cup of low-fat milk, one apple, and cinnamon for breakfast.
- One small banana with two spoonfuls of almond butter for a morning snack

Lunch consists of 2 pieces of whole-wheat bread, 3 ounces of roast beef, 1 teaspoon of horseradish, cucumber slices, and 1 cup of greens.

- Snack in the afternoon: 1 cup sugar snap peas and bell peppers with 1 stick of mozzarella cheese
- Dinner consists of one dish of shrimp and avocado pesto over zucchini noodles.

Day 25

- Two scrambled eggs, two pieces of whole-wheat bread, and one cup of strawberries for breakfast

- One serving of Peanut Butter-Date Energy Balls for breakfast

- Lunch: One dish of shrimp and avocado pesto over zucchini noodles

Snack in the afternoon: 1/2 cup of grapes and one hard-boiled egg.

- Supper is one plate of salad made with spinach and artichokes with parmesan dressing.

Day 26

- Breakfast consists of 1/4 cup granola, 1/4 cup blueberries, and 1 cup plain Greek yogurt.

- One pear and one ounce of cheddar cheese for breakfast - One dish of spinach and artichoke salad with parmesan vinaigrette for lunch

- Snack in the afternoon: 1/4 cup mixed nuts with 1 clementine

- One dish of beef chili in an instant pot with sweet potatoes for dinner.

Day 27

- One dish of muffin-tin mini quiches with spinach and mushrooms for breakfast; one whole-wheat pita bread with half a cup of cherry tomatoes for a morning snack.

- Lunch: One dish of sweet potato and beef chili cooked in an instant pot.

- Snack in the afternoon: 1/4 cup granola, 1/2 cup plain Greek yogurt, and 1/4 cup blueberries The supper consists of one dish of roasted salmon, smoked chickpeas, and greens.

Day 28

- One cup of oatmeal, one cup of low-fat milk, one apple, and cinnamon for breakfast.

- One small banana with two spoonfuls of almond butter for a morning snack

- Lunch consists of one dish of roasted salmon, smoked chickpeas, and greens.

- Snack in the afternoon: 1 cup sugar snap peas and bell peppers with 1 stick of mozzarella cheese

- One dish of brown rice and stir-fried chicken and vegetables for dinner.

Day 29

- Two scrambled eggs, two pieces of whole-wheat bread, and one cup of strawberries for breakfast

- One serving of Peanut Butter-Date Energy Balls for breakfast

- Lunch is one dish of brown rice and stir-fried chicken and vegetables.

Snack in the afternoon: 1/2 cup of grapes and one hard-boiled egg.

- One dish of Mediterranean Quinoa Salad for dinner

Day 30

- Breakfast consists of 1/4 cup granola, 1/4 cup blueberries, and 1 cup plain Greek yogurt.

- One pear and one ounce of cheddar cheese for breakfast

- One dish of Mediterranean Quinoa Salad for lunch

- Snack in the afternoon: 1/4 cup mixed nuts with 1 clementine

- One dish of spaghetti squash spaghetti for dinner

Sugar-free diet recipes

These tasty and simple meals adhere to the no-sugar diet recommendations. More recipes may be found in books or online, or you can make your own utilizing the items that are and aren't permitted on a no-sugar diet. Additionally, you may add additional modifications and swaps for other dietary requirements and preferences, including gluten-free, dairy-free, vegan, or vegetarian.

Shrimp and Avocado Pesto over Zucchini Noodles

Components:

- 4 medium zucchini, thinly sliced or spiralized

- 1/4 cup toasted pine nuts

- 2 ripe avocados, pitted and peeled

- 2 peeled garlic cloves

- 1/4 cup fresh basil leaves

- Half a cup of lemon juice

- 1/4 cup water, as required

- Salt and pepper, to taste

- One pound of big, peeled and deveined shrimp

- Two tsp olive oil

- To taste, red pepper flakes

Guidelines:

- Cook the zucchini noodles in a large pan over medium-high heat for approximately 10 minutes, tossing periodically, until they are crisp but still soft. Empty the surplus liquid and move it to a spacious bowl.

- Toast the pine nuts in a small skillet over medium heat for approximately 5 minutes, shaking the pan often, or until aromatic and brown. Put aside.

- Avocados, garlic, basil, lemon juice, salt, and pepper should all be combined in a food processor or blender and processed until smooth and creamy. As necessary, add more water to change the consistency. Put aside.

- Heat the oil in a second, big pan over medium-high heat. Cook the shrimp for approximately 10 minutes, flipping once, or until they are pink and well-cooked. To taste, add more salt, pepper, and red pepper flakes for seasoning.

- Toss the zucchini noodles with the avocado pesto and sprinkle the pine nuts and prawns over top to serve. Have fun!

Changes and replacements:

- Almonds, walnuts, or pistachios are a few examples of other nuts that may be substituted for pine nuts.

- You may use any kind of fresh herbs, such as parsley, cilantro, or mint, for the basil.
- Any kind of protein, like chicken, beef, tofu, or beans, may be substituted for the shrimp.

Romaine & Artichoke Salad with Parmigiano-Reggiano Dressing

Components:

- 1/4 cup toasted almond slices

- 6 cups baby spinach

- 1 (14-ounce) container drained and chopped artichoke hearts

- 1/4 cup of olive oil;

- 1/4 cup of shredded Parmesan cheese

- One teaspoon Dijon mustard

- Two teaspoons apple cider vinegar

- Toppings of salt and pepper

Guidelines:

- Combine the spinach, almonds, Parmesan cheese, and artichoke hearts in a big salad dish.

- Mix the mustard, vinegar, oil, salt, and pepper in a small container with a tight-fitting cover. Shake well to emulsify.

- Drizzle the salad with the dressing just before serving, tossing to coat. Have fun!

Changes and replacements:

- You may substitute any kind of green, such as kale, arugula, or romaine lettuce, for the spinach.

- You may use any kind of cheese, such as feta, goat, or mozzarella, for Parmesan.

- Almonds may be swapped out for any kind of nut, including pecans, walnuts, and pistachios.

Instant Pot Sweet Potato and Beef Chili

Components:

- One pound of lean ground beef

- One diced onion - Four minced garlic cloves

– Two tsp of chili powder

- One-tsp each of oregano and cumin

- 1/4 teaspoon black pepper

- 1/2 teaspoon salt

One fifteen-ounce can of tomato sauce

One 14.5-oz can of chopped tomatoes;

- one 4-oz tin of green chiles

- One fifteen-ounce can of drained and washed black beans

- Two medium sweet potatoes, peeled and cubed

- 1/4 cup of finely chopped cilantro

- For serving, sour cream, shredded cheese, and green onions (optional)

Guidelines:

- Select the sauté option after turning on the Instant Pot. Add the meat, onion, garlic, cumin, chili powder, oregano, salt, and pepper when the oil has heated.

- Cook for around 15 minutes, breaking up the meat with a wooden spoon, or until it is browned and cooked through. If necessary, drain the extra fat.

- To the Instant Pot, add the sweet potatoes, diced tomatoes, green chilies, tomato sauce, and beef broth. Mix well to blend. Set the valve to sealing, close the lid, and lock it. Set the timer for 15 minutes on high pressure and choose between the manual or pressure cook modes.

- After the cooking period is over, let the pressure fall naturally for ten minutes before cautiously opening the vent valve to discharge the last of the pressure. Remove the top and mix in the cilantro and black beans. Try the seasoning and adjust as needed.

- When ready to serve, spoon the chili into bowls and garnish with cheese, sour cream, and green onions, if preferred. Have fun!

Changes and replacements:

- You may use any kind of ground meat, such as pig, chicken, or turkey, for beef.

- You may substitute any kind of bean, such as kidney, pinto, or white beans, for the black beans.

- Any kind of potato, including white, red, or yellow potatoes, may be substituted for sweet potatoes.

Muffin-Tin Mini Quiches with Spinach and Mushroom

Components:

- Olive oil, one tablespoon

- cooking spray

- One chopped onion

- Two cups of sliced mushrooms

- 6 eggs

- 2 cups baby spinach

- To taste, salt & pepper

– 1/4 cup of skim milk

– 1/4 cup of Parmesan cheese, grated

Guidelines:

- Set an oven temperature of 375°F. Apply cooking spray in a 12-cup muffin tray very lightly.

- In a big pan, heat the oil over medium-high heat.

- Cook the onion and mushrooms, turning occasionally, for approximately 15 minutes, or until they are soft and browned.

- Cook the spinach for a further five minutes, or until it wilts.

- To taste, add salt and pepper for seasoning.

- Combine the eggs, milk, and cheese in a medium-sized bowl; add salt and pepper to taste.

- After dividing the vegetable mixture among the muffin cups equally, cover each cup with approximately 3/4 of the egg mixture.

- Bake until the eggs are firm and brown, 15 to 20 minutes.

- After allowing the quiches to cool somewhat in the pan, release the edges using a knife. Have fun!

Changes and replacements:

- You may substitute any kind of vegetable, such as broccoli, zucchini, peppers, or tomatoes, for the spinach and mushrooms.

- Any kind of cheese, such as cheddar, mozzarella, or feta cheese, may be substituted for Parmesan.

- To increase the protein and taste of the vegetable combination, you may add some cooked bacon, ham, or sausage.

Date Energy Balls with Peanut Butter

Components:

– 1 cup of dates, pitted

- 1/4 cup natural peanut butter

- 1/2 cup rolled oats

- Half a cup of chia seeds

- One-fourth teaspoon of salt

Guidelines:

- Process the dates in a food processor or blender until a sticky paste forms. After transferring, combine the oats, peanut butter, chia seeds, and salt in a big bowl. Toss to fully blend. 16 balls, each approximately an inch in diameter, should be formed out of the dough and put on a baking sheet covered with parchment paper. Chill for a minimum of 60 minutes or until solid. Have fun!

Changes and replacements:

- Dates may be substituted with any kind of dried fruit, such as raisins, figs, or apricots.
- You may use any kind of nut butter, such as cashew, almond, or sunflower seed butter, for peanut butter.
- You may substitute any kind of seed, such as flax, hemp, or sesame seeds, for the chia seeds.

Alright, I'll go on to the chapter on recipes and a meal plan for a sugar-free diet. This concludes the chapter:

Roasted salmon served over greens and smoky chickpeas

Components:

- 2 tablespoons, divided; - 4 (4-ounce) salmon fillets; - Salt and pepper to taste

- Two tablespoons, divided, of smoked paprika

- One fifteen-ounce can of washed and drained chickpeas

- 1/4 cup of freshly chopped parsley

- Half a cup of lemon juice

- Four cups of baby spinach or kale

Guidelines:

- Cover a baking sheet with parchment paper and preheat the oven to 425°F. Add one teaspoon of smoked paprika, salt, and pepper to the fish to season it.

- Transfer to the baking sheet that has been preheated and cover with a tablespoon of oil. Bake the salmon for 15 to 20 minutes, or until it's cooked through and flaky.

-In a big pan, warm the leftover oil over medium-high heat.

- Cook the chickpeas, turning periodically, for approximately 15 minutes, or until they are crisp and brown. Add the remaining smoked paprika and season with salt and pepper. After adding the lemon juice and parsley, turn off the heat.

- Blanch the spinach or kale in a big saucepan of boiling water for approximately two minutes, or until it's wilted and vibrant green. Squeeze and drain any extra water. To serve, split the salad leaves among four plates, then place the chickpea mixture and salmon on top. Have fun!

Changes and replacements:

- You may substitute any kind of fish, such as trout, halibut, or cod, for the salmon.

- You may substitute any kind of green, such as arugula, collard, orchard, for the kale or spinach.

- Any kind of bean, such as kidney, pinto, or white beans, may be substituted for the chickpeas

CONCLUSION

Now that this book is almost over, I hope you have gained a lot of knowledge and liked reading it. Through this book, you have learned:

- What is sugar and why is it bad for your weight, health, and overall well-being?
- How to spot added sugar in food and drink items and substitute it with natural, nutrient-dense options.
- What to eat and avoid while on a no-sugar diet, as well as how to begin and maintain one.
- How to manage sugar cravings and withdrawal symptoms by coming up with workable fixes and coping mechanisms.
- How to stick to a no-sugar diet while dining out, traveling, celebrating, and interacting with others; how to turn a no-sugar diet into a lifestyle rather than a passing trend.

- How to organize and make delectable and simple sugar-free diet meals and dishes, as well as how to enjoy food without added sugar.

You can get a lot of advantages and benefits by eating no sugar, including:

Enhancing your well-being and avoiding or controlling long-term conditions including diabetes, cancer, heart disease, and obesity.
- Improving your vitality, attitude, and mental clarity while lowering tension and anxiety.
- Increasing your awareness of natural tastes, resetting your taste receptors, and savoring your meal more.
- Reducing food waste and temptation while also saving time, money, and energy.
- Achieving your objectives and aspirations and feeling good about yourself.

A sugar-free diet is a lifelong habit rather than a short-term solution. A habit that has the power to improve your life. a routine that might improve your health and happiness. a routine that has the power to improve you as a person.

Nevertheless, it takes time to develop a habit. It requires dedication, time, and work. It requires tolerance, tenacity, and assistance. Not just intention, but action is required.

For this reason, I urge you to act and begin your sugar-free path right now. There's no need to wait until tomorrow, next week, or next month. Never wait for the ideal circumstance, strategy, or inspiration. Don't wait for others to do the task with you or on your behalf.

Simply carry it out. Right now.

Everything you need to be successful is here. You possess the resources, the tools, and the knowledge. You are in charge; you have the option and the duty. You possess the ability, the chance, and the difficulty.

This book is yours.

This book serves as a friend, companion, and guide for you. This book serves as your source of encouragement, inspiration, and support. This book is your accomplishment, your gift, and your prize.

To help you begin and maintain a sugar-free diet, use this book. You can manage your sugar cravings and withdrawal symptoms by using this book. Make a no-sugar diet a way of life, not just a fad, with the aid of this book. Make use of this book to organize and cook sugar-free diet dishes.

Make changes to your life with the aid of this book.

You're capable of it. You can give up sweets. You can survive without sugar.

You can both be well and joyful.

You can be your best self.

You can succeed without sweets.

I'm grateful that you read this book, and I hope your path without sugar is filled with success.